SCIENCE AND NEW MEDICINES
ISSUES OF APPROVAL, ACCESS, AND PRODUCT SAFETY

Daniel E. Harmon

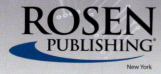
New York

Published in 2009 by The Rosen Publishing Group, Inc.
29 East 21st Street, New York, NY 10010

Copyright © 2009 by The Rosen Publishing Group, Inc.

First Edition

All rights reserved. No part of this book may be reproduced in any form without permission in writing from the publisher, except by a reviewer.

Library of Congress Cataloging-in-Publication Data

Harmon, Daniel E.
New medicines : issues of approval, access, and product safety / Daniel E. Harmon.—1st ed.
    p. cm.—(Science and society)
Includes bibliographical references and index.
ISBN-13: 978-1-4358-5026-2 (library binding)
1. Drugs—Juvenile literature. 2. Drugs—Safety measures—Juvenile literature. 3. Drugs—Law and legislation—Juvenile literature. 4. Drug approval—Juvenile literature. I. Title.
RM301.H36 2009
615'.1—dc22

                                                           2008013696

Manufactured in Malaysia

On the cover: A quality control technician works inside an Illinois laboratory where a blood substitute is being developed. Scientists are researching synthetic substances that might carry oxygen through the circulatory system.

CONTENTS

INTRODUCTION | 4

1 THE ENDLESS WAR—HUMANS VERSUS PHYSICAL AILMENTS | 8

2 PROBLEMS IN MEDICAL PROBLEM SOLVING | 16

3 CONTROLLING THE DRUG INDUSTRY— THE ROLE OF THE FDA | 26

4 BAD MEDICINE | 34

5 WHO SHOULD DECIDE? | 42

GLOSSARY | 50

FOR MORE INFORMATION | 52

FOR FURTHER READING | 55

BIBLIOGRAPHY | 56

INDEX | 61

INTRODUCTION

Medical science is something like war. The bad guys are diseases that can harm or kill the human body and injuries that cause great pain. The good guys are laboratory researchers who constantly seek effective antidotes, cures, and pain remedies. Some observers believe that the scientists are winning in their medical detective work and counterattacks against germs and wounds. Some believe they are losing. Virtually everyone agrees there will never be a complete victory or loss, just a never-ending struggle.

American pharmacists fill more than three billion prescriptions each year, according to pharmaceutical industry estimates. Drugs unquestionably save lives and improve health and the quality of life. On rare occasions, they also harm and kill those who take them. Between those extremes, they produce countless different effects on different people who have different physical, mental, and emotional conditions.

Lab scientists around the world experiment with new medications to combat illnesses and to relieve pain and stress. Most of the new drugs that reach consumers serve those purposes, some more effectively than others. Sometimes, though, people use drugs for the wrong reasons and take larger doses than they should. Sometimes, even when they use them properly, the effects are not entirely good. A drug that relieves pain might damage the liver or dangerously quicken blood circulation. A drug that calms stress might destroy brain cells. A drug that fights cancer might make a body too weak to overcome a common cold.

Medical news reports are alarming. Drugs approved by the U.S. Food and Drug Administration (FDA) are regularly found

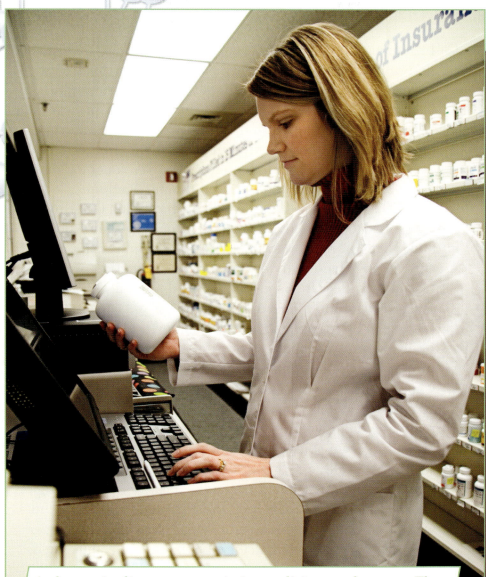

A pharmacist dispenses prescription medicine at a drugstore. The pharmacy is the end point in a distribution system that begins with the drugmaker and includes numerous "middlemen." Inspectors must check regularly for problems that can occur along the way.

to produce unforeseen and dangerous, sometimes deadly, side effects—after years of prescribed use, in some cases. These are just a few examples:

- In January 2008, the FDA cautioned health care providers that antiepileptics, a category of medications for treating such conditions as seizures, bipolar disorder, and migraine headaches, can be dangerous. Over a period of several years, the agency analyzed follow-up study results from the makers of eleven antiepileptics. Four suicides and 105 reports of suicidal tendencies occurred among almost 28,000 test patients who received the medications.
- The FDA warned in February 2008 that Botox (botulinum toxin) had been linked to instances of respiratory failure and other bad reactions, sometimes fatal. Botox is a protein commonly injected under the skin by cosmetic doctors to fill out wrinkles. It has also been used to treat people with muscle disorders. The agency pointed out that nothing seemed to be wrong with Botox itself and that the problems likely occurred because of overdoses and the use of Botox for purposes other than those approved.
- Chattem, Inc., a drug company, in February 2008 voluntarily recalled its Icy Hot Heat Therapy products after receiving reports of first-, second-, and third-degree burns "resulting from consumer use or possible misuse."
- In March 2008, the FDA alerted consumers to adverse effects from misusing Tussionex, a prescription cough medicine made by UCB Inc. The FDA said some patients were taking—and some doctors were prescribing—bigger or more frequent doses than the manufacturer recommended. Such misuse could be fatal.

Those and other problems are why extensive testing is required before a new medication becomes available to the general public. Yet, many people, especially terminally ill patients, do not understand why the FDA seems to drag its feet in approving new medications that offer them hope for a cure. New drug development for children and teens is often also particularly slow.

In one sense, it is a debate over numbers. A clinical test of a medication among a thousand patients might suggest it is effective but results in five severely adverse reactions. Does that mean the drug is too risky? For a simple cough medicine, the answer probably is yes. For a cancer drug, most patients probably would say no—they gladly will take their chances at those odds.

So there is much more to this war than the good of science versus the bad of disease. Within the good army, there is fighting over the quality of the weapons (medications). There is disagreement over the process of developing and distributing the weapons. There is distrust toward drugmakers, government regulators who oversee drug companies, and distributors. There are questions of timing and costs. Some of the medical debates and investigations make little sense to average citizens, but all consumers should be concerned.

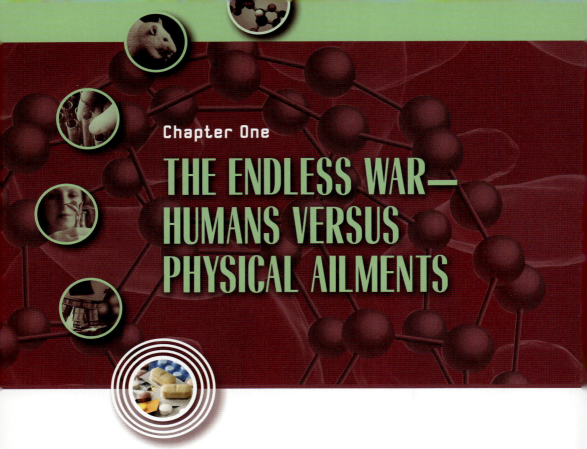

Chapter One
THE ENDLESS WAR—HUMANS VERSUS PHYSICAL AILMENTS

It could be argued that since the beginning of human history, dangerous germs and accidental injuries have been our worst enemies. Almost from the beginning, humans have been looking for remedies. The quest to live longer, active, pain-free lives was as much a part of ancient cultures as it is today.

Medical Treatment in the Past

Ancient peoples believed many of the diseases they suffered were the work of evil spirits. They did not know how to cope. "Doctors" of those days might try mysterious potions and exotic charms to cure or ward off illnesses. Sometimes they literally tried to beat the illness out of the victim's body or to starve the disease (and often the patient). One brutally grotesque measure was trepanning, cutting a hole in the skull to let the evil influence escape from the victim's body.

By about 2500 BCE, certain ancient civilizations were beginning to discover the medicinal qualities of plants. In Egypt, tannic acid from acacia nuts was applied to burns. Castor oil and figs became common laxatives.

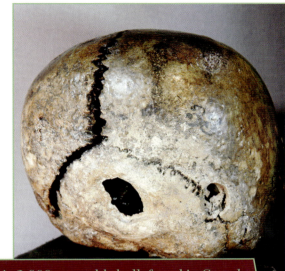

This 2,000-year-old skull, found in Canada, shows the results of trepanning. Trepanning was the cutting of a hole in the skull in hopes of releasing evil, disease-causing spirits.

The Mesopotamians are believed to have created more than five hundred drugs from plants and minerals. In India, certain roots and plants were found useful for blocking pain and treating snakebites. The ancient Greeks were seriously interested in analyzing medical problems. Hippocrates, the Greek physician who lived almost 2,500 years ago, is considered the "father of modern medicine." Among other advances, he advocated preventive medicine.

Medical advances slowly continued in Europe and Arabia during the Middle Ages. Schools of medicine were established in Italy, England, and France.

Overall, however, progress in treating and preventing disease was limited. Doctors of the day proposed and debated strange theories. A leading English physician, for instance, suggested that all diseases resulted from an imbalance in nervous energy.

Modern Medical Research

Not until the late 1800s did chemists and doctors begin to find truly effective (and relatively harmless) medications. Their investigations multiplied and flourished into the twentieth century. The results speak for themselves. In 1900, the average life expectancy in the United States was about forty-seven years. Today, it is approximately seventy-eight years (with women tending to live about seven years longer than men).

In the early decades of modern medical research, fervent doctors, determined to find solutions to health crises, worked on their own. One example was Louis Pasteur, a pioneer in the germ theory of disease causes. Pasteur was a student assistant to one of his Paris medical college professors when he began experimenting with the effect of polarized light on natural and artificial chemical nutrients in the 1840s. He is remembered for his later work in purifying milk from bacteria and helping develop vaccines against rabies and other deadly diseases.

Louis Pasteur (1822–1895) was a renowned French scientist. Among other achievements, he proved germs can cause disease and developed vaccines against such deadly illnesses as rabies.

Today, inquisitive medical scientists can receive financial support for their experiments. A good deal of new drug research is funded by major pharmaceutical companies. As of 2000, the drug industry was spending about $26 billion per year on medical research. Drug companies

THE ENDLESS WAR—HUMANS VERSUS PHYSICAL AILMENTS | 11

have a good reason to invest so much money. New medication sales, if successful, can bring the manufacturer a lot of money.

The government also supports medical research. In particular, the National Institutes of Health (part of the U.S. Department of Health and Human Services) as of 2001 was spending about $20 billion per year on medical research, including new drug development. Typically, the NIH provides research grants to university- and college-based scientists. Private institutes and foundations also support drug research with grants.

Until the late twentieth century, most drug research began with test tube experiments. Now, much of it is being done with computer microchips and other cutting-edge technology. This is possible because of an extraordinary breakthrough in science during the past ten years: the decoding of the human genome,

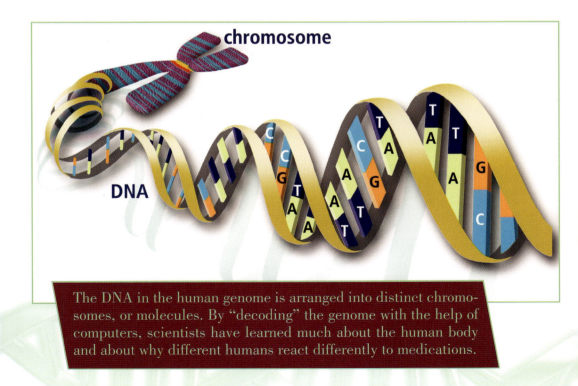

The DNA in the human genome is arranged into distinct chromosomes, or molecules. By "decoding" the genome with the help of computers, scientists have learned much about the human body and about why different humans react differently to medications.

Drugs Are Last Resorts

All doctors need good reasons for prescribing medications. Most drugs are potentially toxic, or poisonous. Some are more dangerous than others. Unless they are needed to help cure or prevent an illness or to help heal an injury, they would not be prescribed at all. Most potential new drugs being examined in test labs today will not be approved by the FDA, even if they show promise in treating certain diseases. The reason is that they may do more harm than good. They might permanently damage the heart, liver, kidneys, brain, or other parts of the body. They can be fatal if used wrongly.

In developing a new medication, scientists must determine to what extent the substance will be more harmful than helpful. The FDA requires that an experimental drug be within an acceptable level of toxicity in multiple preclinical studies before the agency will allow it to even be tested on humans.

If the new drug eventually makes it to market, it likely will be labeled with precautions. People with certain health conditions, particularly heart, liver, or respiratory problems, may be advised not to take it.

or gene structure. Computers can help scientists analyze the genetics of humans and identify defective genes that may make a person susceptible to particular diseases. Drugs thus can be developed that precisely target the problem gene(s), rather than treat the disease globally and less specifically. Such targeted therapies can also minimize "side effect" damage to healthy cells. The study of genetics takes disease fighting to a fascinating inner molecular level.

Fighting Illnesses with Poisons

There are two general kinds of diseases: infectious and noninfectious. Infectious illnesses are caused by microorganisms and can often be transmitted from one human to another (the flu is an example). Noninfectious diseases range from arthritis to heart disease to cancer.

Both types of diseases can be treated. Ironically, the drugs used to treat them both usually contain substances that are alien to the human body—poisons. Diseases do not occur naturally in humans, and neither do the remedies.

Just as in days of old, modern scientists find valuable uses for poisonous substances. Snake and insect venom, for example, are ingredients in some vaccines. Vaccines are developed to make people immune to the harmful effects of the poisons. Scientists have found other beneficial characteristics of certain poisons. An example is Capoten, used to treat patients with high blood pressure; it was derived from the poison of a South American viper. Of course, such substances must be prepared and tested exhaustively before the public can be allowed to take them.

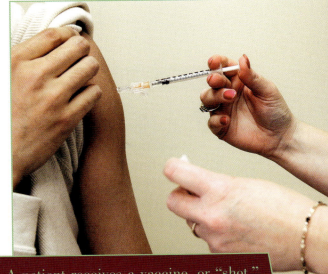

A patient receives a vaccine, or "shot." This inoculation is part of testing for an experimental flu vaccine. Researchers want to know if the medication can prevent a deadly form of avian flu.

Most drugs today are synthetics, or chemical creations. They do not occur naturally, but are made to resemble natural chemicals. The reason medical scientists prefer them is that they are easier to control than natural chemicals. Regardless of their makeup, they are foreign objects to the human body. The lab scientists who develop them and physicians who prescribe them to fight an illness must consider their possible negative effects.

When initial research suggests that a new substance may be useful for medical treatment, scientists begin an extensive testing process. First, the substance is tested on small animals, then on larger ones. Scientists observe both the helpful and harmful effects it produces. If the results point to a possibly valuable new treatment with minor risks, they apply for permission to try it on volunteer human patients.

That is just the beginning of the testing program. It will probably be a long time before the drug is approved for sale to the public. Amazingly, only about 1 percent of all drugs in research testing will ever be approved for general use.

MYTHS AND FACTS

MYTH If a medication can be bought over the counter at a drugstore, it must be safe. It's been tested strictly and meets government requirements.

FACT Keep an eye on FDA medication alerts and drug recall notices. Although all over-the-counter items must be FDA-approved, problems frequently arise with old and new medications. Pay special attention to the precautions on the label. A medication that works wonders for one individual might be dangerous for someone who has certain health conditions or is taking other medications at the same time.

THE ENDLESS WAR—HUMANS VERSUS PHYSICAL AILMENTS

MYTH If a doctor prescribes it, it obviously is safe to use.

FACT Sadly, not all doctors carefully examine the patient's medical history and take into account other medications the patient might be taking—medications that might make for a nasty drug combination. (This may be the patient's fault for not reporting such details to the doctor. It is particularly important to tell the doctor about all medicines that you are taking, including herbs and supplements.) Furthermore, not every patient responds to the same medication in the same way. Adverse side effects should be reported immediately to the doctor.

MYTH Cancer is incurable.

FACT Most forms of cancer can be counteracted and slowed, to some extent, by medication. Cancers in children and teens are far more treatable and curable than they are in adults. Results vary from patient to patient, but with chemotherapy, radiation, or surgery, many types of cancer—including some of the most critical—have been eradicated and have not recurred. Researchers continually seek new medications to combat specific forms of cancer. They have scored remarkable successes in recent years.

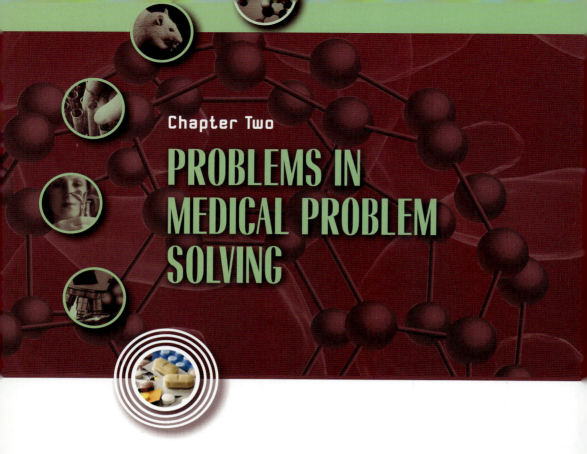

Chapter Two
PROBLEMS IN MEDICAL PROBLEM SOLVING

The health care industry is one of the largest moneymakers in America. It is also one of the largest employers. From major cities to small towns, workers at many levels, from delivery and clerical personnel to doctors and nurses to research scientists, contribute to society and earn their livings in the medical service field. They, like everyone else, sometimes make mistakes. A few of them tell white lies or commit outright crimes.

When something goes wrong in medical treatment, patients and their families—and the press, and politicians, and government officials whose careers might be affected by the fallout—demand explanations. They want to be able to attach blame to someone or to some company or regulatory organization. That may be no simple matter. Confusing and complex issues are often involved.

Safety: A Long-Term Concern

The first question consumers ask about a new medication is: how safe is it? In some cases, the answer may not become clear for many years. An infamous example of long-term results is diethylstilbestrol (DES). Approved by the FDA in the 1940s, it was commonly prescribed for pregnant women for more than thirty years. Its purpose was to improve the health of unborn babies and help prevent miscarriages.

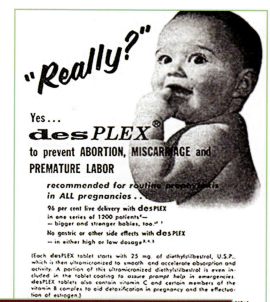

A 1957 medical journal advertisement promotes desPLEX for pregnant women. The drug, recommended for safer pregnancies and healthier babies, later was shown to cause health problems.

Problems with DES began to be reported in the 1960s. Of more than five million Americans exposed to DES over the years, many—including prenatal patients and their now-adult children—have suffered adverse effects. Problems include breast, vaginal, and prostate cancer; infertility; reproductive injuries; and immune system disorders. The FDA in 1971 warned doctors not to prescribe it for pregnant patients, but the drug was not banned.

On the other hand, many people wonder why the FDA seems to be holding up the approval of potential wonder drugs. Dr. Stanislaw Burzynski, a Polish-born doctor practicing in Houston,

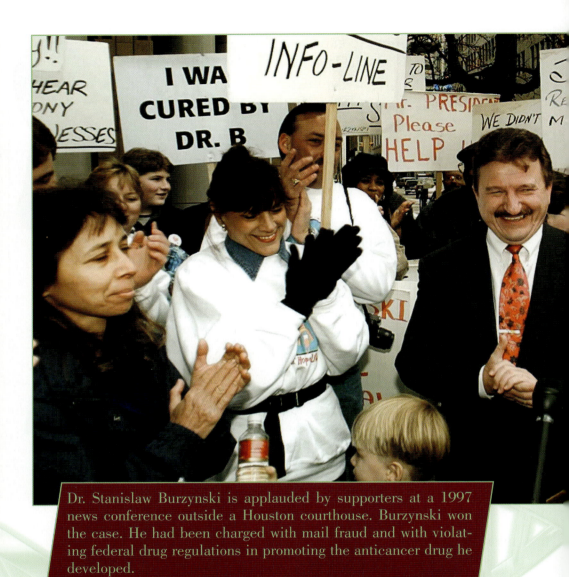

Dr. Stanislaw Burzynski is applauded by supporters at a 1997 news conference outside a Houston courthouse. Burzynski won the case. He had been charged with mail fraud and with violating federal drug regulations in promoting the anticancer drug he developed.

Texas, developed a peptide he named antineoplaston during the 1970s. The word "antineoplaston" literally means "anticancer." The doctor claims success in treating certain cancer tumors that resisted all other medications.

PROBLEMS IN MEDICAL PROBLEM SOLVING

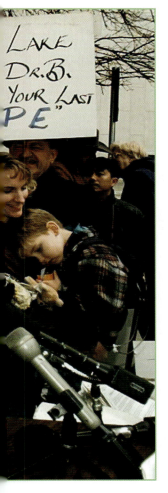

Burzynski did not partner with any large pharmaceutical company in testing and processing his treatment but developed it himself. Beginning in 1983, the FDA repeatedly blocked his attempts to bring the drug to market. On several occasions the agency sought legal action against him. In 1997, he was tried for interstate commerce of an unapproved drug, insurance fraud, and contempt of court. Burzynski survived the court challenges, but he has been frustrated in trying to obtain FDA approval for testing and marketing his medications.

Some observers believe Burzynski's maverick approach may have needled both FDA officials and the medical establishment. Skeptics in the medical community say the overall effectiveness of Burzynski's treatments has never been proved. Some have called him a quack doctor and questioned both the effectiveness and safety of the drugs he promotes. Hundreds of patients, meanwhile, call him a hero and say they owe him their lives.

The FDA in 2004 gave Burzynski "orphan drug" status for some of his anticancer medications. This classification encourages drug development for the treatment of life-threatening illnesses. Clinical trials are ongoing at this time.

A New Safety Dilemma: Counterfeit Medicine

A growing concern today is drug counterfeiting. Doctors prescribe legitimate medications, and pharmacists dispense what they think are legitimate medications. Still, patients do not always get what they think they are getting. The culprit is not the pharmacist or the doctor who prescribed the drug. It is a "gray market of middlemen," according to medical reporter Katherine Eban, author of a book titled *Dangerous Doses*. From the time a product leaves a drug company's manufacturing facility until it arrives in pharmacies, many people handle it. On rare occasions, middlemen have been charged with altering approved medications or making substitutions. Some have put false labels on the drugs.

Why? To make more money. If, for example, they claim the drug is many times its actual strength, they can charge much more for it than it is worth. Eban reported that a third of the licensed wholesale drug companies in Florida were suspected of dealing improperly. Wholesalers are go-betweens, buying large quantities of medications from drug manufacturers, then distributing and selling them to drugstore chains, independent pharmacies, hospitals, and clinics. In some distribution channels, as many as a dozen individuals process the medication from the time it leaves the manufacturer until a patient buys it. In some channels, dishonest workers have infiltrated the system.

Can't the U.S. Food and Drug Administration put a stop to such fraud? Not directly. The FDA regulates drugmakers, not wholesalers. Law enforcement and health officials in each state are responsible for policing that link in the distribution chain.

A few pharmacists have been convicted of stealing portions of expensive medicines from their own businesses to sell on the black market. They mix the remaining portions—the medicine left on their shelves, which they will dispense to customers—with worthless ingredients to make up the difference. This can endanger critically ill patients because they are not receiving as much pure medication as they need.

Although certain drug middlemen, pharmacists, and doctors have resorted to counterfeiting and counterfeit medication sales, many other medical and pharmaceutical professionals have been victimized. Thieves, often agents of organized crime, have broken into wholesale warehouses, drugstores, and hospitals to steal medications.

No one can be sure how much of the medication being dispensed today is counterfeit. Estimates have ranged from less than 1 percent to as much as 10 percent. The racket is growing because, since medicine is very expensive, it can be quite profitable. For people who know how the drug supply chain works, it isn't a difficult form of fraud to carry out. (Medications, though, can be tested in a pharmaceutical laboratory to determine the bogus ingredient and its concentration if a counterfeit medication is suspected.)

The Ethics of Medical Research

"Medical ethics (bioethics)" is a modern-day term. It encompasses several concerns that did not seem to occur to most doctors and scientists of old. For example,

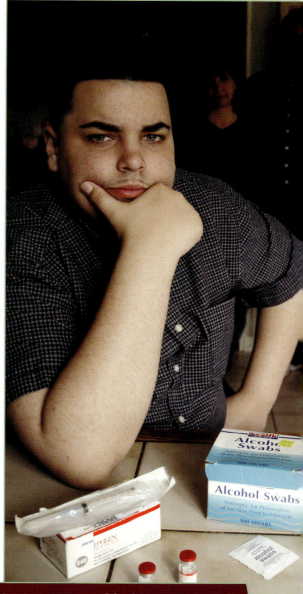

This sixteen-year-old of Deer Park, New York, was a victim of counterfeit medication. After undergoing surgery to replace his liver, the teen took the false drug expecting it to help him heal.

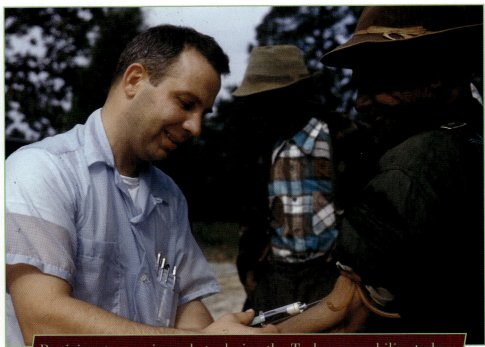

Participants are given shots during the Tuskegee syphilis study. The project, carried out over a period of years, involved sharecroppers in Alabama. It became highly controversial after it was revealed that doctors in the study withheld penicillin treatment from the test patients.

people now consider it unethical to deceive patients to get them to participate in medical experiments. In the past, that was not the case. Ethical questions also are raised in such far-flung matters as a doctor's role in treating a patient (What if the patient's disease places the doctor at risk?), birth control recommendations, and the burden of health care costs as the American population ages.

In medical research, a notorious example of bad ethics was the Tuskegee syphilis study of the mid-twentieth century. Black sharecroppers in Alabama were recruited for a clinical study of syphilis, a sexually transmitted disease, over a period of years. They were not fully informed of what they were doing and were

Testing New Drugs on the Poor

After pharmaceutical companies obtain FDA approval to test new drugs on humans, they must find human patients. Many volunteers are healthy individuals ("controls") for some medications or vaccines, while others are frail patients with chronic diseases who have not been helped by any approved medications and thus are willing to try a possible new cure even if it is risky.

For American drug companies, finding clinical volunteers is not easy. Fewer than 5 percent of Americans are willing to participate in testing, according to CenterWatch, a medical information provider. Many are physically unable. Some tests require that patients live at or near the testing location for weeks or months, and few patients can afford to do that. Others are simply afraid of the dangers.

Part of the solution to the volunteer shortage, drug companies have found in recent years, is to engage patients in third world countries. American companies have set up clinics on several continents, in nations where clinical codes and requirements are not as strict as they are in the United States. There have been accusations (which may or may not be merited) that some of the test participants are not aware they are receiving experimental medication.

In her book *The Body Hunters*, journalist Sonia Shah questions the ethics of overseas testing. Even though the testing is legal, it is not being done for the purpose of helping poor people in those countries. In effect, it uses them to make sure a drug is safe—a drug that will mainly benefit more well-off patients in the United States and other developed nations. Many trial subjects overseas, Shah says, face "an impossible choice—be experimented on or die for lack of medicine—that undermines human rights."

Those who disagree see the practice as an opportunity, not an impossible choice, for poor test subjects.

not given proper clinical care. Even after penicillin, an effective syphilis cure, became a common treatment, research doctors withheld it from the Tuskegee patients. The doctors wanted to continue their observations of syphilis's long-term effects on the human body, leaving the patients untreated and often with devastating complications to the nervous system.

Critics of the modern approach to medical research say it is unfair. Medical research in wealthy countries, including the United States, is focused on treating diseases that are common in those countries. In undeveloped countries, meanwhile, millions of people are dying of diseases such as malaria, which are not serious problems in richer nations. The governments of poor countries cannot afford to pay for extensive medical research to end those diseases.

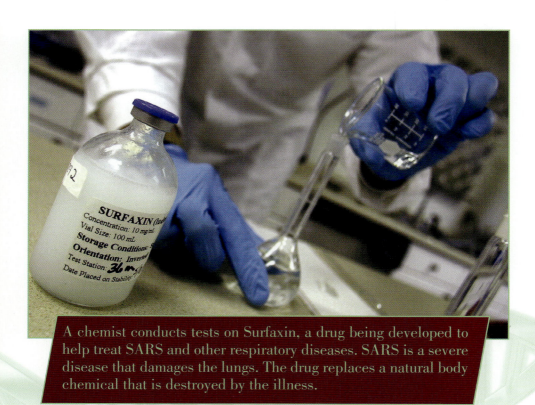

A chemist conducts tests on Surfaxin, a drug being developed to help treat SARS and other respiratory diseases. SARS is a severe disease that damages the lungs. The drug replaces a natural body chemical that is destroyed by the illness.

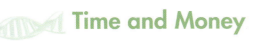 Time and Money

In the United States, the drug approval process is so demanding and time-consuming that only large drug companies or specially funded researchers can afford to develop new medications. Estimates vary, but most sources agree it takes several years and costs drug developers several hundred million dollars, on average, to pass all the hurdles, from discovery of a medication to consumer use. In 2007, the Pharmaceutical Research and Manufacturers of America estimated it costs approximately a billion dollars and takes almost fifteen years to move a new medication from discovery to pharmacy counters.

To save money, even large drug companies are increasingly going out of the country to conduct patient testing. The cost of clinics and hospitals for patient trials is much less in poorer countries. It also costs less to recruit patients in large foreign cities with millions of people in desperate need of medical help.

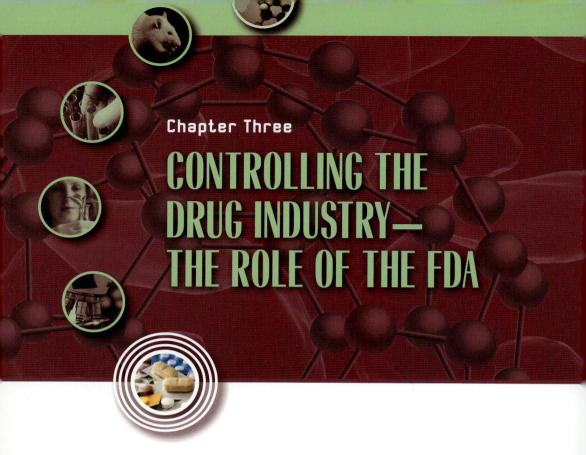

Chapter Three

CONTROLLING THE DRUG INDUSTRY—THE ROLE OF THE FDA

Americans depend on the U.S. Food and Drug Administration for drug safety. The FDA is part of the U.S. Department of Health and Human Services. Its basic role is to enforce the Federal Food, Drug, and Cosmetic Act (FD&C Act), passed in 1938. Since then, the agency has been given responsibility for enforcing almost fifty FD&C amendments and additional laws.

The FDA's mission is to protect the public health by ensuring the safety, effectiveness, and quality of food and drug products. Both new and existing medications and medical devices are among the items the FDA regulates. Its authority is not absolute, though. For example, it does not actually carry out the extensive testing processes that are required for

CONTROLLING THE DRUG INDUSTRY—THE ROLE OF THE FDA

new medications. Rather, it analyzes test results that are submitted to it by lab scientists, some of them hired by drug companies, who perform the tests. Once it approves a new medication for public use, the FDA makes sure its labeling is correct and advertising is not misleading, and conducts inspections. It has little control over the product's distribution channels—the transportation and delivery system through which medication shipments get from the factory to the consumer. In this and other areas of the drug industry, mischief and mistakes are known to occur. The FDA itself has been called to task for mishandling applications and failing to hold pharmaceutical companies fully accountable for the safety and effectiveness of products they sell.

> MedWatch (www.fda.gov/medwatch) is a service of the FDA that provides drug safety alerts and product information. Doctors and patients can report suspected problems with medications.

Offices within the FDA include the Center for Drug Evaluation and Research (CDER), National Center for Toxicological Research, Center for Biologics Evaluation and Research, Center for Devices and Radiological Health, Center for Veterinary Medicine, and Center for Food Safety and Applied Nutrition. The Center for Drug Evaluation and Research is primarily responsible for ensuring that Americans have access to drugs that are safe and effective. Its medical professionals examine applications for new medications and determine their outcomes. Meanwhile, they monitor the more than ten thousand drugs being sold in the United States. They also watch for false claims in drug advertising.

The sheer number of different drugs on the market and in development creates an enormous task for the CDER. FDA officials say the agency does not have enough staff or funds to safeguard food and drug consumers adequately. To fully ensure drug safety, the agency would need many more people spending more time evaluating new drugs and monitoring existing ones.

The FDA's Drug Approval Process

A pharmaceutical company might scrutinize thousands of new chemical compounds before it identifies a combination that it believes is worth marketing. When it does, it first tests the medication on animals. If animal testing suggests that the medication may be useful (and not too harmful), it applies to the FDA for permission to continue its tests on human volunteers.

When a new medication is approved for human testing, it must be observed through several test stages. Phase I studies usually include twenty to eighty healthy volunteer patients (but may have fewer patients for some trials of new medicines, such as chemotherapies). For certain medications, including those intended for cancer treatment, Phase I participants may be terminal patients who are willing to try a possible remedy and accept possible risks. The studies must show that the drug's toxicity is within acceptable levels. Many approved drugs—both prescription and over-the-counter medicines—cause harmful side effects, from nausea and hypertension to hair loss. The issue is how much good they can accomplish, in balance with how much harm they might cause.

If a new drug passes Phase I, testing advances to Phase II. Here, the drug is administered to a larger test group. Researchers study more closely the drug's possible effectiveness in treating specific medical conditions or diseases, as well as the shorter-term side effects the drug might produce.

U.S. Drug Regulation: A Capsule History

More than two hundred years ago, Congress created the Marine Hospital Service to aid sick and disabled sailors. This was at a point in American history when the fledgling navy held the key to national security. In 1912, this became the U.S. Public Health Service, later transformed into the U.S. Department of Health and Human Services. The Food and Drug Administration was established to enforce the Food, Drug, and Cosmetic Act of 1938.

What became the FDA's Center for Drug Evaluation and Research began separately in 1906. One official in what was then the Federal Bureau of Chemistry was assigned to look into problems with medications that were on the market at the time.

Phase III tests might involve a thousand or more participants. Researchers may use two or more test groups to determine how the new medication compares with existing treatments. "Control groups" are given the standard-of-care existing medications (or possibly a placebo medication, depending on the medication being tested and the goal of the trial). Scientists already know what effects the control group treatments are likely to produce. The "treatment group," meanwhile, receives the experimental mediation. At the end of the testing, results are compared. Such studies may be "blinded" so that the participants and/or researchers do not know which medication a patient is receiving until the study is completed.

Some drugs during the early testing stages show potential for treating life-threatening diseases for which there are no known cures. The FDA may grant them "accelerated development/review" status—the "fast track" toward approval. The agency also tries to make what it calls "treatment investigational new drugs" available as soon as possible to terminally ill patients who have no other treatments available.

Experimental medications for cancer and AIDS typically have received fast-track status. The FDA permitted prescriptions of interleukin-2, an experimental cancer drug, for terminal patients in 1987 even before the drugmaker formally sought approval. AIDS—originally a killer disease—has become manageable during the last decade with the use of a new class of drugs called protease inhibitors. Scientists continue to search for new AIDS/HIV medications that are more effective and produce fewer negative side effects.

Continuing Uncertainties

Regardless of clinical testing, it is virtually impossible to know what a medication's long-term effects might have on certain patients. It is one thing to introduce a new chemical or chemical compound into the human body and observe the results. It is another to determine what effects that chemical may produce if certain other chemicals are present in the body. When different chemical substances mix, things can become very dicey. Drug A may be completely beneficial when taken by itself. Drug B likewise may be useful and harmless when taken alone. But if the two are taken together, their interaction inside the body can be fatal.

Scientists generally know which classes of drugs are unsafe to mix. Because people use thousands of different medications, though, there is no way for a drug company to test all the possible combinations with a new trial drug. If the drug earns FDA approval and goes on the market, it could be years before complications arise and can be studied and understood.

The FDA in May 2008 announced a new program called the Sentinel Initiative. It provides early monitoring of the effects of

CONTROLLING THE DRUG INDUSTRY—THE ROLE OF THE FDA

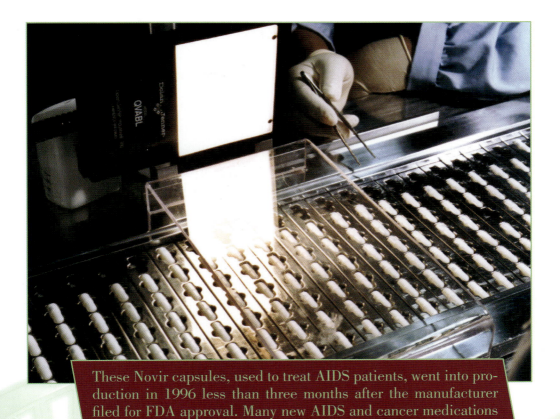

These Novir capsules, used to treat AIDS patients, went into production in 1996 less than three months after the manufacturer filed for FDA approval. Many new AIDS and cancer medications get "fast track" status to shorten the approval process.

new medications on patients. Officials examine Medicare claims, looking for potential risks associated with drugs. In the past, for the most part, the FDA had to wait for patients, doctors, or drug companies to report problems. Their information was inconsistent. One person may have considered an adverse drug effect to be very serious; another may have accepted it as a necessary downside of treatment. By using Medicare data, officials can see how many patients taking a particular drug report similar bad reactions.

The problem of medical troubleshooting is complicated by variations in individuals' health. A drug or combination of drugs may be harmless to most consumers but may cause serious

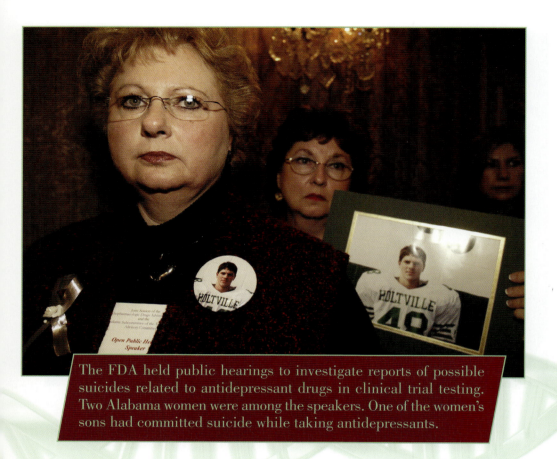

The FDA held public hearings to investigate reports of possible suicides related to antidepressant drugs in clinical trial testing. Two Alabama women were among the speakers. One of the women's sons had committed suicide while taking antidepressants.

problems for someone with asthma, high blood pressure, diabetes, or a psychological disorder. In some cases, doctors are unsure why a medication is safe for most people but harmful for a few individuals. Antifloxacin, an antibiotic introduced in the early 1990s, is prescribed to treat various symptoms ranging from eye inflammation to pneumonia to sexually transmitted diseases. For most patients, it does what it is supposed to do. Some people who take it experience diarrhea, dizziness, and other adverse side effects. In extremely rare cases, patients have suffered permanent damage, with recurring fits of psychosis.

Medications for Sale Online

It would be difficult enough for a government watchdog agency to cope with medications that pass through regular distribution channels. In the new era of the Internet, the FDA also has to keep watch over medications that are marketed online. Millions of Americans have begun shopping online for everything from clothes to cars. Internet shopping for medications is appealing for several reasons. For one, it's easy; shoppers can find what they want and place their orders quickly, without leaving their computer desks. They can have products delivered to their homes overnight, if they wish. Second, they can often find lower prices online than they do in drugstores.

There is a third incentive. On the Internet, patients might find medications that are unavailable from American pharmacies. These include drugs still in testing. The FDA cautions consumers against buying such products.

In March 2008, the agency announced it had sent warning letters to a foreign individual and six American companies for selling drugs online that allegedly treat or prevent sexually transmitted diseases. In some cases, advertisers claimed their products could do what approved medications could not do. Other marketers falsely indicated their products were approved by the FDA. Dr. Janet Woodcock, acting director of the FDA Center for Drug Evaluation and Research at the time, said, "The products pose a serious health threat to unsuspecting consumers who don't know that these products are not FDA-approved and have not been proven safe or effective."

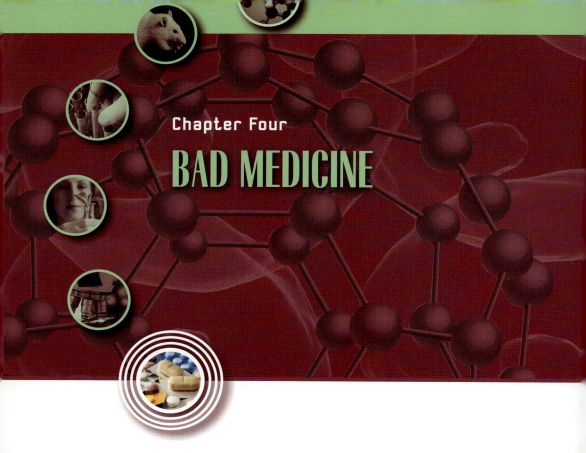

Chapter Four
BAD MEDICINE

Vioxx, an analgesic drug produced by Merck & Co., Inc., was approved by the FDA in 1999 for treating arthritis. Prescribed widely, it was used by more than eighty million patients in eighty countries. Five years later, Merck voluntarily recalled the drug after extensive tests indicated it could cause cardiovascular problems. The complications usually did not become apparent until more than a year after patients began the treatment.

The FDA was criticized for not banning the drug sooner because Vioxx for several years had been suspected of a link to heart problems. Instead of ordering it off the market, the FDA, shortly before the Merck decision, actually had expanded

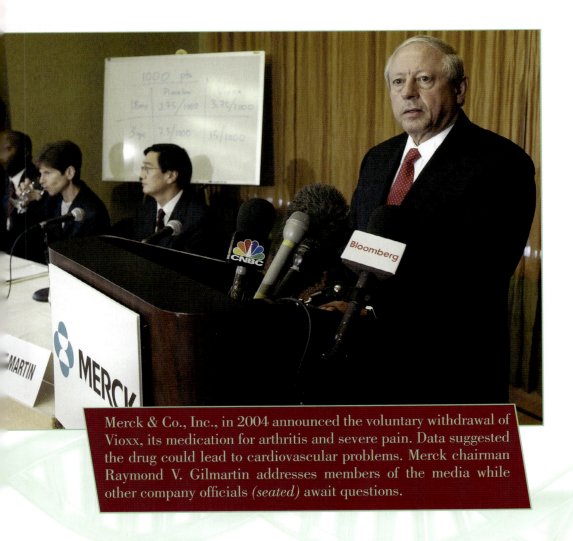

Merck & Co., Inc., in 2004 announced the voluntary withdrawal of Vioxx, its medication for arthritis and severe pain. Data suggested the drug could lead to cardiovascular problems. Merck chairman Raymond V. Gilmartin addresses members of the media while other company officials *(seated)* await questions.

its approved use to include the treatment of juvenile rheumatoid arthritis. Earlier in 2004, the agency had approved it for treating migraine headaches.

Vioxx is one of many recent examples of medications being pulled from pharmacy shelves after follow-up trials, wider and longer use, and customer complaints reveal bad side effects. Critics of the FDA often cite these cases as evidence the administration is doing a poor job of safeguarding the public health.

Cholesterol and Diet Drugs

Statins are a controversial group of medications prescribed to improve cholesterol levels, which in turn reduces the risk of strokes and heart attacks. An early product in the drug class, Baycol, was withdrawn from the market in 2001. But several statins have become best-selling medications since the late 1990s. Lipitor led all U.S. drug sales by 2004; Zocor ranked second. Lipitor sales in 2007 totaled almost $13 billion. A newer, more powerful statin, Crestor, was introduced in 2003, and within a year Public Citizen, a health research group, was calling for its removal. Crestor had already been linked to about thirty cases of severe kidney problems, although it is quite effective at lowering cholesterol. The FDA in 2005 issued an alert that Crestor and other statins might cause muscle damage and kidney failure, but it did not order them off the market. These medications are very effective, but doctors also counsel patients seriously about the rare, but dangerous, side effects. Doctors and patients must monitor closely for early signs of these side effects.

Pfizer Inc., the maker of Lipitor, came under fire from Congress in February 2008 for its advertising campaign to promote the drug. A TV commercial showed Dr. Richard Jarvik, a noted heart researcher and endorser of Lipitor, rowing a scull across a lake. It was revealed that Jarvik does not row; the rower in the ad was a stunt double. Pfizer announced it would scrap the commercial. The incident raised questions about the ethics of advertising prescription medications. Some doctors believe prescription medication advertisements can be misleading and should be banned. They point out that the medicines are unnecessary for many patients, and they can be overly expensive.

Fen-phen was a weight-loss drug popular in the 1990s. It was banned in 1997 after indications that it could damage heart valves. Some users since then have claimed the drug caused them permanent heart damage.

BAD MEDICINE | 37

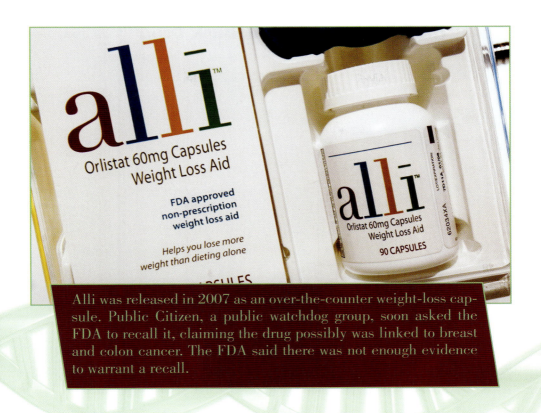

Alli was released in 2007 as an over-the-counter weight-loss capsule. Public Citizen, a public watchdog group, soon asked the FDA to recall it, claiming the drug possibly was linked to breast and colon cancer. The FDA said there was not enough evidence to warrant a recall.

Alli (Xenical), a diet drug made by GlaxoSmithKline, was challenged by Public Citizen in 2007 for its alleged potential to cause colon and breast cancer. Although the watchdog group asked the FDA to order its recall, the administration said there was no conclusive evidence linking Alli to cancer.

In February 2008, Palo Alto Labs voluntarily recalled Aspire36 and Aspire Lite, two of its diet supplement products. The company did so after FDA lab studies showed that the products contained trace elements of sulfoaildenafil, a substance that causes blood vessels to dilate. This chemical can cause dangerously low blood pressure if taken by people who are also taking nitrate medications. Nitrates are commonly prescribed for people with heart problems, diabetes, and high cholesterol levels. The incident was another example of how certain medications might

Thalidomide: A "Comeback Drug"

In the early 1960s, thalidomide was prescribed to pregnant women in different countries to ease morning sickness and help them sleep. Soon after its release, in many cases, children were born with shrunken arms or legs, or with no limbs at all. Thalidomide was determined to be the culprit.

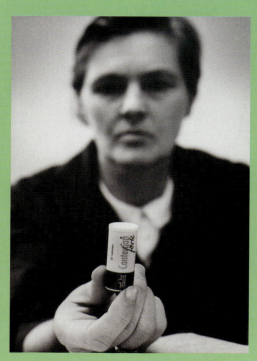

Dr. Frances O. Kelsey was the FDA doctor who delayed approval of thalidomide in the 1960s. Approved in Europe, the drug was linked to thousands of infant deformities.

Interestingly, the FDA never approved the drug for public release in the United States, thanks to a suspicious agency doctor who processed the thalidomide application from an American drug company, Richardson-Merrell Inc. Despite pressure from the drugmaker to approve the medication quickly, the FDA delayed the process. A growing public outcry from Europe then spelled doom for thalidomide, a drug that had injured approximately fifteen thousand infants.

Even more interesting, scientists in recent years have found that thalidomide is in fact a valuable medication, but not for its original intent. It can help treat people with certain types of cancer, immune system disorders, and rheumatoid arthritis. It now is approved by the FDA for those purposes.

be safe if taken alone but can lead to trouble for some individuals if taken in combination with other substances.

More Recalls

Baxter International Inc., in early 2008, recalled its heparin products and stopped producing the blood thinner. Some patients who used heparin experienced numerous adverse effects. These included vomiting and other digestive disorders, chest pain, low blood pressure, fast heart rate, fainting, skin irritations, and bleeding tendencies. In some cases, the symptoms were severe. Baxter initially reported the problems and began a partial recall in January 2008 but did not order a complete recall until more than a month later. The FDA explained that Baxter's heparin brand was used widely in operating rooms and kidney dialysis centers, and that to remove it all at once would have created major problems at those facilities. By late February, the FDA said other suppliers of blood thinners were able to meet the needs of medical centers, and Baxter withdrew the remaining supplies.

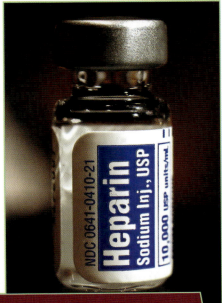

Heparin, a blood thinner, in 2008 was withdrawn from hospitals and medical centers by Baxter International Inc. The medication was linked to circulatory and digestive disorders as well as skin irritations.

Able Laboratories, Inc., a New Jersey–based maker of several dozen medications including generic pain relievers and heart and blood pressure drugs, recalled all of its products and closed its operations in 2005. The move—one of the largest drug recalls in U.S. history—followed reports that it failed to ensure satisfactory quality control and submitted questionable lab test reports to the Food and Drug Administration. The FDA noted that Able withheld unfavorable test data.

Pet medicine is also subject to FDA regulation, and it, like human drugs, sometimes turns out to be harmful. In November 2007 and March 2008, the Hartz Mountain Corporation recalled shipments of Hartz Vitamin Care for Cats. FDA sampling indicated the vitamin lots may have been contaminated by *Salmonella*. *Salmonella* is a bacterium that can cause digestive disorders in cats and humans (often from food poisoning). At the time it withdrew the vitamins, Hartz said it had received no reports of actual sickness related to the incident, either in animals or humans.

Gray Areas of Medication Monitoring

Some health alerts have been difficult to analyze. During the 1980s and 1990s, certain FDA-approved medications for correcting irregular heartbeats came under fire. Thousands of patients were dying because of the drugs that were supposed to help them, critics claimed. The FDA responded that the medications had been approved for patients with specific heart conditions and that some doctors were prescribing them for patients with different symptoms. The agency pointed out that it has no control over medical practice; doctors can prescribe approved medications to patients as they see fit.

In monitoring medications, the FDA often identifies potential problems that are not serious enough to warrant recalling the products. It issues safety information alerts and instructs the drug companies to revise their product labels. One recent example involved Tamiflu, a flu treatment. The FDA received reports from Japan and elsewhere that some patients taking Tamiflu experienced delirium and bizarre behavior that caused injuries. Although no positive connection had been established between the drug and the incidents of abnormal behavior, the drugmaker,

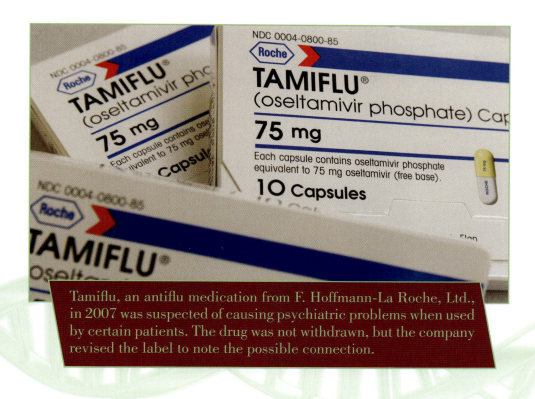

Tamiflu, an antiflu medication from F. Hoffmann-La Roche, Ltd., in 2007 was suspected of causing psychiatric problems when used by certain patients. The drug was not withdrawn, but the company revised the label to note the possible connection.

F. Hoffmann-La Roche, Ltd., revised its label to note the possible association.

The FDA provides MedWatch, an information resource and voluntary problem-reporting program. MedWatch invites consumers and health professionals to report adverse reactions, concerns with the quality of medications, and errors in the use of products. Its regular alerts describe possible problems with drugs, dietary supplements, medical devices, and biological products.

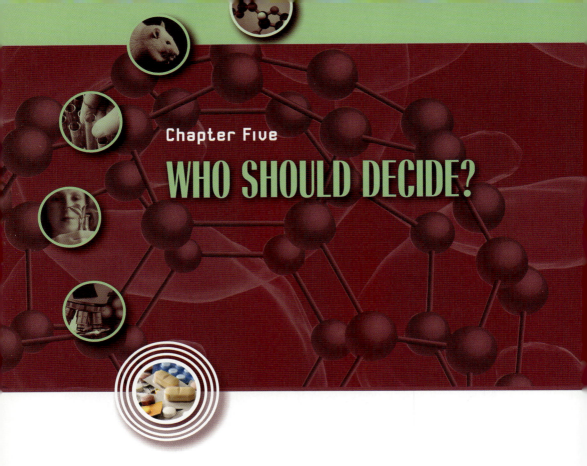

Chapter Five
WHO SHOULD DECIDE?

"It's my life. Choosing medications should be my decision." That argument is not uncommon among people suffering from terminal or unbearably painful diseases and physical conditions. They reason that no bad side effects of an experimental drug can be worse than what they are experiencing. They eagerly would try unapproved medications, if they could obtain them.

Is the U.S. Food and Drug Administration too controlling? Too slack? Is it always working in the best interests of American citizens? Or does it sometimes allow drug companies to get away with development and testing practices that could place lives in jeopardy?

A Question of Trust

Ketek (telithromycin) is an antibiotic used to fight pneumonia, sinusitis, and bronchitis. The FDA approved it in 2004. In 2006, the FDA received reports of Ketek patients who suffered liver failure; several deaths were linked to the drug. The agency eventually responded by restricting the drug's use to patients suffering from life-threatening pneumonia.

In early 2008, some congressional representatives were pressing the FDA to turn over to them documents related to the Ketek case. They suspected that when the FDA approved the medication, agency officials knew that much of the testing data was unreliable and might have been manipulated. According to a report by the Associated Press in 2006, U.S. senator Charles Grassley voiced concern over "the cozy relationship between some drug companies and the Food and Drug Administration."

The Ketek controversy was one of many in recent years that have raised questions about the performance of the FDA. The 2005 resignation of FDA commissioner Lester Crawford was just one more sign, in the opinion of critics, that the agency is alarmingly influenced by food and drug companies. It was revealed that Crawford held stocks in companies that sold medical devices,

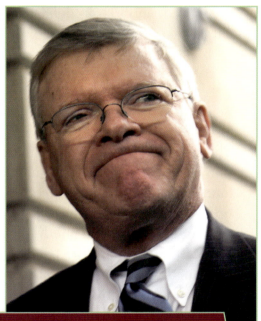

Lester Crawford resigned his post as FDA commissioner in 2005. A year later, he pleaded guilty to federal charges of conflict of interest and false reporting.

foods, and beverages. A year after his resignation, Crawford pleaded guilty in a federal magistrate court to conflict of interest and false reporting. Owning those stocks was illegal for Crawford because the companies were regulated by the agency he headed.

Agency detractors for years have claimed that the FDA sometimes turns a blind eye to questionable drug and food industry activities, endangering the safety of citizens. At the same time, former agency employees have reported that the FDA retaliates against drug companies if they complain to congressional representatives or the news media about the way the FDA handles the approval and inspection process.

The FDA responds that it is doing the best it can with the limited budget (about $2 billion) and personnel (about nine thousand employees) it has available. Approved medications are continually monitored, and FDA officials caution that even regulated products carry risks.

Medical Patients Go on Vacation

Some desperately sick Americans are looking to Asia, Europe, and elsewhere for treatment that is unavailable in the United States. The Chinese biotechnology industry has drawn particular attention for producing medications and gene therapy programs not found in other countries. The world's first gene therapy medication, Gendicine, was developed in China for treating certain types of cancer. American medical professionals are wary, though, noting that clinical drug trials are not required in China.

Americans also are buying FDA-approved medications overseas, where they are less expensive. The Food and Drug Administration has cautioned Americans against foreign drug purchases. One reason is a confusion in brand names. For example, the U.S. drug Norpramin is used to treat depression; a Spanish drug by the same name is used to treat stomach ulcers.

Many Americans—not just fatally ill patients—travel to other countries for medical and surgical procedures because

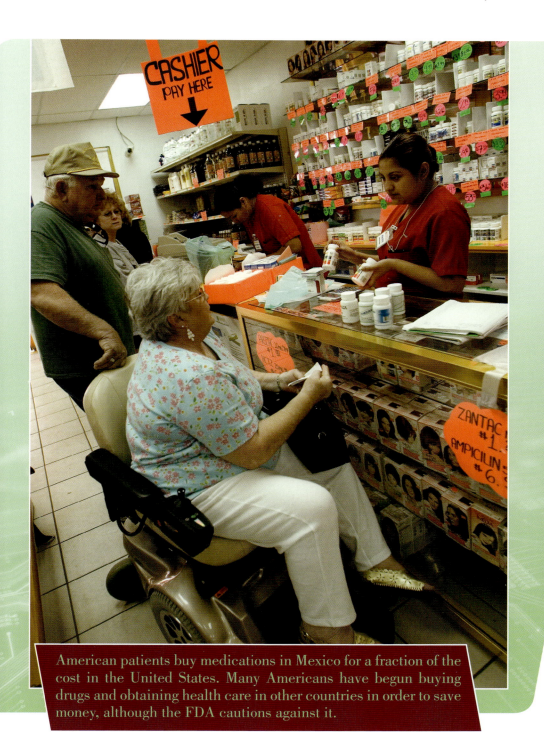

American patients buy medications in Mexico for a fraction of the cost in the United States. Many Americans have begun buying drugs and obtaining health care in other countries in order to save money, although the FDA cautions against it.

Medical Tourism

A new travel industry dubbed medical tourism has emerged in recent years. Internet-based companies such as Healthbase (http://www.healthbase.com) and Treatment Abroad (http://www.treatmentabroad.net) help Americans find internationally accredited medical facilities in Asia, India, Mexico, Turkey, and other countries. They say the treatment outcomes abroad generally are as satisfactory as those in the United States and in some cases are better. Some five hundred thousand Americans went overseas for medical treatment in 2005, according to the National Coalition on Health Care.

The growth in medical tourism and medication purchases abroad raises questions not only about America's drug and treatment approval processes, but about its overall health care system. Why, for instance, can people in those parts of the world buy certain medications before they are approved in the United States? And why are drugs, medical care, and health insurance substantially more expensive in this country?

they are so much cheaper there. American patients may undergo minor surgery such as root canals, cataract correction, and cosmetic repairs, as well as hip and knee replacements and major heart and spinal operations. Overseas medical care is especially appealing to Americans who are underinsured or uninsured and who cannot afford the rising cost of health coverage. If a dental or eye operation would cost thousands of dollars in the United States, but can be performed elsewhere by a well-qualified doctor for several hundred dollars, the savings would pay for the trip. Some American businesses and even insurance companies are looking into "outsourcing" the medical care of their employees and customers.

Prescriptions, Power, and Politics

Monitoring the U.S. drug industry is a complex challenge for the FDA and for nongovernment medical watchdog organizations. Regulators do not always see eye to eye with powerful, well-financed drug companies or with patients clamoring for more effective medications.

The issues also become political. Are drug companies buying favorable influence from elected government officeholders and appointed agency officials? If so, are they doing it legally or illicitly? It is one thing for the pharmaceutical industry to lobby for its causes. Lobbying is part of the American way of life. Countless lobbyists in Washington and in state capitals work to persuade

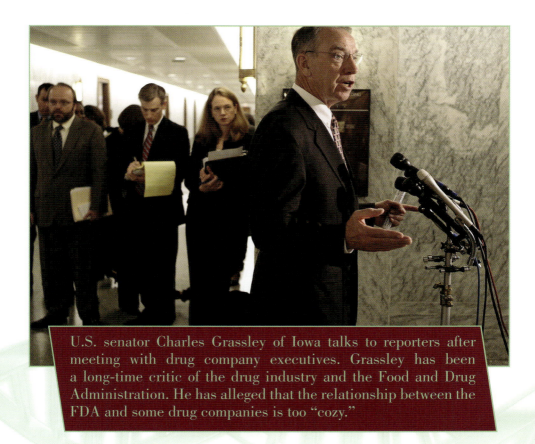

U.S. senator Charles Grassley of Iowa talks to reporters after meeting with drug company executives. Grassley has been a long-time critic of the drug industry and the Food and Drug Administration. He has alleged that the relationship between the FDA and some drug companies is too "cozy."

lawmakers to support their interests. It is different, though, if agents of a drug company pay government officials to rush through an application for a new medication or pay them to ignore certain test results that might alarm medical professionals.

Conclusion

Since the founding of the nation, Americans have based their lives on the idea of freedom. To this day, they are leery of the government's involvement in their lives. In areas where they recognize that government organization and regulation is necessary—such as drug safety—they expect flawless, uncorrupt performance by the government agencies in charge. Yet, all people, including doctors, scientists, pharmacists, and elected and appointed officials, are human. Wherever power is at play, corruption lurks and mistakes are unavoidable.

The U.S. Food and Drug Administration is at the center of a medical debate that probably can never be resolved. On one hand, the agency is under pressure to approve new medications more quickly, especially when it seems possible that cutting-edge drugs might help terminally ill patients. Since the early 1990s, the FDA has reduced its average review and approval time by almost half, from approximately two years to one. (That does not include the time it takes drug companies to test their new products *before* submitting applications to the FDA.) In 2007, by order of Congress, the agency began creating a new drug research center, funded by drug companies, to streamline the development and approval process for new drugs.

Still, the agency's medical professionals and administrators know they will be condemned if a drug they approve later turns out to be more dangerous than the public is willing to accept. Some critics say the approval process does not move fast enough, that the FDA should accelerate its fast track in certain categories. Others contend that the agency should take more time to ensure that drug developers complete exhaustive, accurate testing before any new drug is released. In fairness to the FDA, it should be remembered that in some cases, the side effects of a dangerous drug have not come to light until many years after the drug was approved for marketing. How many years should scientists, drug companies, FDA officials, and doctors wait and see before the testing ends and they can introduce a new medication, concluding that it is safe to use?

Patients and doctors, scientists and drugmakers, politicians and the press constantly examine the pharmaceutical industry and judge the performance of regulatory agencies. While they do, the quest continues for the next miracle drug. Perhaps it will be only a few years—or months—until cures are announced for cancer, heart disease, diabetes, Alzheimer's, arthritis, and other tragic conditions.

GLOSSARY

antibiotic Chemical substance that can cure infections by killing the harmful bacteria.
antidote Medication taken to counteract the negative effects of a specific poison.
biotechnology Science of changing organisms to make them stronger or more useful for certain purposes.
black market Illegal buying and selling of goods.
cardiovascular Related to the heart, blood vessels, and circulation.
cataract A clouding of the eye lens.
chemical compound Substance formed by combining two or more chemicals.
chemotherapy Treatment of cancer and other illnesses with medications.
clinical Type of testing in which doctors study patients' reactions to medications.
consumer A person who buys or uses products.
counterfeiting Making a fake medication or mixing it with a cheap substance to produce greater, but weakened, quantities of it.
dialysis Clinical process for removing poisons and waste matter from the blood of patients with kidney diseases.
dilate To widen or enlarge.
ethics A system of values and moral standards.
generic A usually less-expensive version of a medication that has no brand name.
hypertension High blood pressure.
immune Safe from being affected by a particular disease.
lobbyist A person or group that tries to influence lawmakers on behalf of a special interest.

microorganism A living being so small it can be seen only with a microscope.

over-the-counter Medications that can be sold in retail stores without a doctor's prescription.

peptide A string of amino acids that comprises a small protein.

pharmaceutical Having to do with medications.

placebo A medication that produces no effect; it can be given to a control group in clinical testing for the purpose of comparison with experimental medications.

prenatal Before birth; type of medication or care given to pregnant mothers.

protease inhibitor A type of medication used to treat HIV.

psychosis A mental disorder characterized by a loss of contact with reality and an inability to think clearly.

radiation A form of treatment for certain diseases and conditions, notably cancer.

respiratory Pertaining to the nose, nasal passages, lungs, and other parts of the body involved in the breathing process.

synthetics Drugs created in a laboratory that are a combination of chemical substances.

toxic Poisonous.

toxicity The degree of harm caused by a substance.

toxin A poison produced by a living organism, especially bacteria, capable of causing disease and stimulating the production within the body of antibodies to counter the effects.

vaccine A medication given to a healthy person for the purpose of preventing a specific disease.

wholesaler A person or company that buys large quantities of goods from a manufacturer and sells them to retail stores at a higher price.

FOR MORE INFORMATION

Centers for Disease Control and Prevention
U.S. Department of Health and Human Services
1600 Clifton Road
Atlanta, GA 30333
(404) 498-1515
Web site: http://www.cdc.gov
The CDC provides online information about all types of diseases
    and medical conditions.

Health Canada
Brooke Claxton Building, Tunney's Pasture
Postal Locator: 0906C
Ottawa, ON K1A 0K9
Canada
Web site: http://www.hc-sc.gc.ca/ahc-asc/index_e.html
Health Canada is Canada's federal department responsible
    for health concerns. See especially the "Drugs and Health
    Products" section of its Web site (http://www.hc-sc.gc.ca/
    dhp-mps/index_e.html).

Healthology
500 Seventh Avenue, 14th Floor
New York, NY 10018
Web site: http://www.healthology.com
Founded by two physicians, Healthology distributes doctor-
    generated health and medical information, including articles
    and videos.

National Coalition on Health Care
1200 G Street NW, Suite 250
Washington, DC 20005

(202) 638-7151
Web site: http://www.nchc.org
A nonprofit alliance dedicated to improving health care in the United States.

National Institutes of Health
U.S. Department of Health and Human Services
9000 Rockville Pike
Bethesda, MD 20892
(301) 496-4000
Web site: http://www.nih.gov
The NIH is the primary government agency for conducting and supporting medical research.

National Library of Medicine
8600 Rockville Pike
Bethesda, MD 20894
(888) 346-3656
Web site: http://www.nlm.nih.gov
"The world's largest biomedical library" is part of the National Institutes of Health. Its MedLine Plus Web site provides information about drugs, supplements, and herbs.

New Medications for Kids
About.com: Pediatrics
The New York Times Company
620 Eighth Avenue
New York, NY 10018
(212) 556-1234
Web site: http://pediatrics.about.com/od/childhoodmedications/a/05_new_meds.htm
Information about new medicines that are developed to be more appealing to children. The page is part of About.com's "Health" section (http://www.about.com/health). About.com is a consumer health Web site.

Public Health Agency of Canada
130 Colonnade Road
A.L. 6501H
Ottawa, ON K1A 0K9
Canada
Web site: http://www.phac-aspc.gc.ca
The agency's mission is "to promote and protect the health of Canadians through leadership, partnership, innovation, and action in public health."

U.S. Food and Drug Administration
U.S. Department of Health and Human Services
5600 Fishers Lane
Rockville, MD 20857-0001
(888) 463-6332
Web site: http://www.fda.gov
The FDA publishes information on all food and drug regulation. See especially the Web section for the FDA Center for Drug Evaluation and Research (http://www.fda.gov/cder/index.html) and its page on the new drug development process (http://www.fda.gov/cder/handbook/develop.htm).

Web Sites

Due to the changing nature of Internet links, Rosen Publishing has developed an online list of Web sites related to the subject of this book. This site is updated regularly. Please use this link to access the list:

http://www.rosenlinks.com/sas/medi

FOR FURTHER READING

Fitzhugh, Karla. *Prescription Drug Abuse* (What's the Deal?). Portsmouth, NH: Heinemann, 2005.

Harmon, Daniel E. *The Food and Drug Administration* (Your Government: How It Works). Philadelphia, PA: Chelsea House Publishers, 2002.

Hiber, Amanda. *Are Americans Overmedicated?* (At Issues). Farmington Hills, MI: Greenhaven Press, 2006.

Townsend, John. *Pills, Powders & Potions: A History of Medications* (A Painful History of Medicine). Chicago, IL: Raintree, 2006.

Tuttle, Cheryl Gerson. *Medications: The Ultimate Teen Guide* (It Happened to Me). Lanham, MD: The Scarecrow Press, Inc., 2004.

BIBLIOGRAPHY

About.com: Arthritis. "Vioxx Recalled by Merck Worldwide." September 30, 2004. Retrieved March 28, 2008 (http://arthritis.about.com/od/vioxx/a/vioxxrecall.htm).

Alonso-Zaldivar, Ricardo. "FDA Rules Expand Human Drug Testing." *Seattle Times*, January 13, 2006. Retrieved March 2008 (http://seattletimes.nwsource.com/html/nationworld/2002736983_fda13.html).

Asia Times. "Experimental Drugs Flourish in China." January 9, 2008. Retrieved March 2008 (http://www.atimes.com/atimes/China_Business/JA09Cb02.html).

Brazell, Robert. "Major Drug Maker Recalls Entire Inventory." NBC News, May 31, 2005. Retrieved March 2008 (http://www.msnbc.msn.com/id/8050556).

Bridges, Andrew. "Ex-FDA Chief Pleads Guilty in Stock Case." *Washington Post*, October 17, 2006. Retrieved March 2008 (http://www.washingtonpost.com/wp-dyn/content/article/2006/10/17/AR2006101700573.html).

Cohen, Jay S. "The Truth About Crestor." MedicationSense.com. Retrieved March 2008 (http://www.medicationsense.com/articles/july_sept_04/crestor_truth.html).

Dallas Morning News. "Senate Confirms Bush's FDA Nominee After Filibuster Broken." December 7, 2006. Retrieved March 28, 2008 (http://www.dallasnews.com/sharedcontent/dws/news/nation/stories/120806dnnatfda.2eaedc5.html).

DES Action USA. "DES." Retrieved June 5, 2008 (http://www.desaction.org/aboutdes.htm).

Dooley, Joseph F., and Marian Betancourt. *The Coming Cancer Breakthroughs: What You Need to Know About the Latest Cancer Treatment Options*. New York, NY: Kensington Books, 2002.

Drennan, Kathleen B. "Pharma WANTS YOU: Clinical Trials Are Agencies' New Proving Ground." PharmExec.com,

April 1, 2003. Retrieved March 28, 2008 (http://pharmexec.findpharma.com/pharmexec/PE+Features/Pharma-WANTS-YOU/ArticleLong/Article/detail/53002).

Eban, Katherine. *Dangerous Doses: How Counterfeiters Are Contaminating America's Drug Supply*. Orlando, FL: Harcourt, Inc., 2005.

Elias, Thomas D. *The Burzynski Breakthrough*. Nevada City, CA: Lexikos, 2001.

FDA News. "FDA Alerts Health Care Providers to Risk of Suicidal Thoughts and Behavior with Antiepileptic Medications." January 31, 2008. Retrieved March 2008 (http://www.fda.gov/bbs/topics/NEWS/2008/NEW01786.html).

FDA News. "FDA Issues Alert on Tussionex, a Long-Lasting Prescription Cough Medicine Containing Hydrocodone." March 11, 2008. Retrieved March 2008 (http://www.fda.gov/bbs/topics/NEWS/2008/NEW01805.html).

FDA News. "FDA Notifies Public of Adverse Reactions Linked to Botox Use." February 8, 2008. Retrieved March 2008 (http://www.fda.gov/bbs/topics/NEWS/2008/NEW01796.html).

FDA News. "FDA Warns Companies Importing and Marketing Drugs Over the Internet That Fraudulently Claim to Prevent and Treat STDs." March 6, 2008. Retrieved March 2008 (http://www.fda.gov/bbs/topics/NEWS/2008/NEW01803.html).

Fiore, Marrecca. "Group: Diet Drug Alli Linked to Colon Cancer." FoxNews.com, June 14, 2007. Retrieved March 2008 (http://www.foxnews.com/story/0,2933,282617,00.html).

Green, Saul. "Stanislaw Burzynski and 'Antineoplastons.'" Quackwatch, revised November 21, 2006. Retrieved March 2008 (http://www.quackwatch.com/01QuackeryRelatedTopics/Cancer/burzynski1.html).

Harris, Gardiner. "F.D.A. to Expand Scrutiny of Risks From Drugs After They're Approved for Sale." *New York Times*, May 23, 2008. Retrieved May 23, 2008 (http://www.nytimes.com/2008/05/23/washington/23fda.html).

Hilts, Philip J. *Protecting America's Health: The FDA, Business, and One Hundred Years of Regulation.* New York, NY: Alfred A. Knopf, 2003.

Kaisernetwork.org. "Cost of New Drug Development Reaches $897M, Study Says." May 15, 2003. Retrieved March 2008 (http://www.kaisernetwork.org/daily_reports/rep_index.cfm?DR_ID=17747).

Medical Procedure News. "U.S. Companies Consider Overseas Medical Treatment for Employees." November 6, 2006. Retrieved March 28, 2008 (http://www.news-medical.net/?id=20878).

Microsoft Student 2008. "Drug." CD-ROM, 2007.

MSN.com. "House Panel to Subpoena FDA Officials." January 29, 2008. Retrieved January 30, 2008 (http://news.moneycentral.msn.com/ticker/article.aspx?Feed=AP&Date=20080129&ID=8102227&Symbol=SNY).

MSNBC.com. "New FDA Drug Center Raises Ethical Questions." October 14, 2007. Retrieved March 2008 (http://www.msnbc.msn.com/id/21298130).

Perrone, Matthew. "Democrats Threaten to Hold Bush Official in Contempt Over Sanofi Drug Probe." Yahoo! Finance, February 12, 2008. Retrieved March 28, 2008 (http://biz.yahoo.com/ap/080212/sanofi_congress_hearing.html?v=2).

Saul, Stephanie. "Pfizer to End Lipitor Ads by Jarvik." *New York Times*, February 26, 2008. Retrieved March 28, 2008 (http://www.nytimes.com/2008/02/26/business/26pfizer.html).

Schmit, Julie. "Costs, Regulations Move More Drug Tests Outside USA." *USA Today*, May 16, 2005. Retrieved March 28, 2008 (http://www.usatoday.com/news/health/2005-05-16-drug-trials-usat_x.htm).

Schmit, Julie. "FDA Report Says Able Labs Fudged Drug Tests." *USA Today*, July 12, 2005. Retrieved March 28, 2008 (http://www.usatoday.com/money/industries/health/drugs/2005-07-12-fda-drugs-usat_x.htm).

ScienceDaily. "Solving the US Drug Price Crisis, Experts Propose Solution." March 17, 2008. Retrieved March 27, 2008 (http://www.sciencedaily.com/releases/2008/03/080317105101.htm).

Shah, Sonia. *The Body Hunters: Testing New Drugs on the World's Poorest Patients*. New York, NY: The New Press, 2006.

Sikorski, Robert, and Richard Peters. "Medicine." Microsoft Student 2008 CD-ROM, 2007.

Taylor, Phil. "End of the Line Looms for Able Laboratories." in-Pharma Technologist.com, August 17, 2005. Retrieved March 27, 2008 (http://www.in-pharmatechnologist.com/news/ng.asp?id=61928-able-laboratories-quality-control-liquidation).

U.S. Food and Drug Administration. "Baxter to Proceed with Recall of Remaining Heparin Sodium Vial Products." FDA press release, February 28, 2008. Retrieved March 2008 (http://www.fda.gov/oc/po/firmrecalls/baxter02_08.html).

U.S. Food and Drug Administration. "Chattem Issues URGENT Voluntary Nationwide Recall of Icy Hot Heat Therapy Products." FDA press release, February 8, 2008. Retrieved March 2008 (http://www.fda.gov/oc/po/firmrecalls/chattem02_08.html).

U.S. Food and Drug Administration. "The Hartz Mountain Corporation Recalls Vitamin Care for Cats Because of Possible Health Risk." FDA press release, March 7, 2008. Retrieved March 28, 2008 (http://www.fda.gov/oc/po/firmrecalls/hartz03_08.html).

U.S. Food and Drug Administation. "Palo Alto Labs Issues a Voluntary Recall of Aspire36 and Aspire Lite, Two Products Marketed as Dietary Supplements." FDA press release, February 28, 2008. Retrieved March 2008 (http://www.fda.gov/oc/po/firmrecalls/paloalto02_08.html).

Wolfe, Sidney M. "Letter of concern to Lester Crawford, acting director of the FDA, regarding Crestor, October 29, 2004." Public Citizen. Retrieved March 27, 2008 (http://www.

citizen.org/publications/release.cfm?ID=7341&secID=1668&catID=126).

Zuger, Abigail. "Drug Pitchman: Actor, Doctor or Pfizer's Option." *New York Times*, March 4, 2008. Retrieved March 28, 2008 (http://www.nytimes.com/2008/03/04/health/views/04essa.html).

INDEX

A

Able Laboratories, Inc., 39–40
advertising new medicines
　ethics of, 36
　false claims in, 28, 33
　misleading, 27, 36
AIDS/HIV, 30
Alli, 37
antiepileptics, 6
Antifloxacin, 32

B

Baxter International, Inc., 39
black market, 20
blood thinners, 39
Body Hunters, The, 23
Botox, 6
Burzynski, Stanislaw, 17–19

C

Capoten, 13
Center for Drug Evaluation and Research, 27–28, 29, 33
CenterWatch, 23
Chattem, Inc., 6
Chinese biotechnology industry, 44
Crawford, Lester, 43–44
Crestor, 36
critics, of medical research, 24

D

Dangerous Doses, 20
DES, 17
diet drugs, 36–37

diseases, infectious vs. noninfectious, 13
drug combinations, dangers of, 14, 15, 30, 31–32, 37
drug counterfeiting, 19–21
drugs, unapproved uses of, 6, 40

E

Eban, Katherine, 20

F

Federal Food, Drug, and Cosmetic Act, 26, 29
Fen-phen, 36
F. Hoffmann-La Roche, Ltd., 41

G

gene therapy, 44
genes/genetics, 11–12
GlaxoSmithKline, 37
Grassley, Charles, 43

H

Hartz Mountain Corporation, 40
health care industry, 16, 46
Hippocrates, 9
human genome, 11

I

Icy Hot Heat Therapy, 6
interleukin-2, 30

J

Jarvik, Richard, 36

K
Ketek, 43

L
Lipitor, 36
lobbying/lobbyists, 47–48

M
medical ethics, 21–24
medical tourism
   reasons for, 44, 46
   risks of, 44, 46
Medicare, 31
medicines, poisonous effects of, 12, 28
MedWatch, 41
Merck & Co., Inc., 34
middlemen, 20

N
National Institutes of Health (NIH), 11
new medicines
   and animal testing, 14, 28
   approval process of, 6–7, 14, 19, 28–30, 48
   blind studies of, 29
   and clinical testing, 7, 22–24, 28–30
   and consumers, 6, 7, 17, 27, 28, 31, 33, 41
   and control groups, 29
   distributors/distribution of, 7, 20
   and fast track, 30, 48
   and human testing, overseas, 23, 25
   and human testing, phases of, 28–30
   labels/labeling of, 12, 14, 27
   online distribution of, 33
   side effects of, 4, 6, 7, 12, 14, 15, 17, 28, 30, 31–32, 34–37, 39, 40, 41, 49
   time and cost of testing, 25
   and treatment groups, 29
   treatment investigational of, 30

O
orphan drugs, 19
over-the-counter medications, 14

P
Palo Alto Labs, 37
Pasteur, Louis, 10
pet medicine, FDA regulation of, 40
Pfizer, Inc., 36
pharmaceutical industry/companies
   and funding for drug research, 10
   and overseas research, 23, 25
   political influence of, 43, 47–48
   recalls and, 36–37, 39–40
Pharmaceutical Research and Manufacturers of America (PhRMA), 25
pharmacists, as victims of counterfeiting, 20–21
poisons, as medicines, 13
protease inhibitors, 30
Public Citizen, 36, 37

R
recalls, drug, 34–37, 39–40

S
safety alerts, 6, 14, 40, 41
Sentinel Initiative, 30–31
Shah, Sonia, 23
statins, 36
synthetic drugs, 13–14

T
thalidomide, 38

trepanning, 9
Tuskegee syphilis study, 22, 24
Tussionex, 6

U

UCB, Inc., 6
U.S. Department of Health and Human Services (HHS), 11, 26, 29
U.S. Food and Drug Administration (FDA)
  basic role of, 26
  criticism of, 7, 27, 34, 35, 40, 42, 43–44, 48–49
  lack of staff and funds, 28, 44
  limits of regulatory authority, 20, 26, 27, 40
  offices within, 27
  over-the-counter medications and, 14
  Stanislaw Burzynski and, 17, 19

V

Vioxx, 34–35

W

wholesalers, 20
Woodcock, Janet, 33

About the Author
Daniel E. Harmon is the author of more than sixty books and a veteran periodicals editor and writer whose articles have appeared in many national and regional magazines and newspapers. His educational books include volumes on the U.S. Food and Drug Administration and four volumes on psychological disorders and their medical treatment. He lives in Spartanburg, South Carolina.

Photo Credits
Cover Tim Boyle/Getty Images; cover (bottom inset) © www.istockphoto.com/Marcelo Wain; cover and interior background and decorative elements © www.istockphoto.com/Sebastian Kaulitzki, © www.istockphoto.com/Yuri Khristich; © www.istockphoto.com/appleuzr, © www.istockphoto.com/marc brown, © www.istockphoto.com/bigredlynx; p. 5 © www.istockphoto.com/Sean Locke; p. 9 Werner Forman/Art Resource, NY; p. 10 Library of Congress Prints and Photographs Division; p. 11 U.S. Department of Energy Genome Programs, http://genomics.energy.gov; p. 13 Alex Wong/Getty Images; p. 17 Courtesy DES Action, http://www.desaction.org; pp. 18–19, 21, 31, 32, 39, 43 © AP Images; p. 22 NARA, Southeast Region, Record Group 442, Tuskegee Syphilis Study Administrative Records 1929–1972; p. 24 William Thomas Cain/Getty Images; p. 35 Stan Honda/AFP/Getty Images; p. 37 Chris Hondros/Getty Images; p. 38 Art Rickerby/Time & Life Pictures/Getty Images; p. 41 Justin Sullivan/Getty Images; p. 45 Radhika Chalasani/Getty Images; p. 47 Chip Somodevilla/Getty Images.

Designer: Evelyn Horovicz; Cover Designer: Nelson Sá
Editor: Kathy Kuhtz Campbell